POWER
ISO-BOW
ISOMETRIC
Method

POWER ISO-BOW ISOMETRIC

Method

The Best Isometric Exercises that build muscle, increase POWER, with the Isometric Power Pulse Method

BECOME A ISO-BOW MAN!

The Power Iso-Bow Isometric Method was written to help you get closer to your physical potential when it comes to real muscle sculpting strengthening exercises. The exercises and routines in this book are quite demanding, so consult your physician and have a physical exam taken prior to the start of this exercise program. Proceed with the suggested exercises and information at your own risk. The Publishers and author shall not be liable or responsible for any loss, injury, or damage allegedly arising from the information or suggestions in this book.

Power Iso-Bow Isometric Method
muscle-building Course

By

Birch Tree Publishing
Published by Birch Tree Publishing

Birch Tree Publishing

Dedication

For Popeye Spinach **POWER AND STRENGTH**, focus on **ISOMETRICS!**

Contents

BUILD "ISOMETRIC" POWER

Introducing Isometric Pulses the worlds fastest strength, fat-loss producing system EVER!

Introduction by John Hughes

I have been involved with athletics all of my life, from college wrestling to World Championship Master's Wrestling in my 60s. Coupled with over 15 years of high school coaching, I have always strived for top physical performance in strength and flexibility for myself and the athletes I coached. I purchased my first Bullworker in the 1960s and was impressed with how quickly my body responded to Bullworker strength training. The portability of the product meant I never had to get rid of it due to space restraints and over the next 30 years, the ability to supplement any exercise routine with a quick Bullworker workout, always complimented my desired fitness goal.

In 1999, I became the North American distributor for Bullworker and began to work on design changes to make the product much more challenging, yet always maintaining the portability aspect of this time tested and proven fitness product. In recognizing the importance of cross-training principles for maximum fitness results, I designed additional products that kept with the Bullworker portability concept with each product able to be used either separately or combined for maximum fitness results in a complete cross-training program.

In 2010, I purchased most of the Global rights to Bullworker and have reintroduced Bullworker training principles that have been effective since 1962 and resulted in over 10 million units sold. Proven as the ultimate portable fitness products, Bullworker continues to deliver results to everyone, any age, wherever they exercise.

Today, I present the Bullworker Isometric Power Series. This book is about transforming your body, mind and spirit, which is what health, strength and physique enhancement is all about. I am really excited and positive to say that once you try the programs in this book, you will make some of the best gains you've ever made.
Join the men and women that are already using The Bullworker Isometric Power Series and programs with great success. **GET TRANSFORMED** today.

Keep pulling and pushing

Yours in Strength and Power

John Hughes

An open letter by Marlon Birch
DEVELOP POWERFUL MUSCLES NOW

9/DEVELOP POWERFUL MUSCLES NOW

Isometric exercises trigger as much chiseled muscle growth and strength in quick, no-time-wasted bursts. It is the fastest way of stimulating as much muscle growth as possible within a short space of time. How? With the new Power Iso-Bow Isometric Method which proves that my "efficient workouts" can help you activate significantly more lean growth fibers—and build muscle much faster with effective Isometric Power-Pulses Mega-Power-Growth phases.

You will use quick, effective Isometric routines for every targeted muscle in your exercise program— each time. These Power-Growth workouts will allow optimal recovery time to keep you progressing threefold. The full programs are spectacular at triggering serious strength gains with workouts that get the muscle-sculpting job done in double quick time.

As most readers know, I've been doing Isometric exercises for over 30 years. So when it comes to results and effective training programs, which will make you work each muscle from one or two specific positions to ensure optimum-muscle-activation. The Power Iso-bow Isometric power-phases are extremely effective.

However, I've made it even better and faster based on my experimentation and research. It's the perfect solution to a condensed program, making it even more efficient at increasing lean, ripped to the bone muscles.
Practice and consistency is the name of the game here for self mastery.

Progress takes time; and each day of pleasant practice you will automatically see a huge difference. You will, however, gain control over your muscles and increase your strength and physique tremendously. Daily you will feel and see the strength gains and physique changes, day by day and week by week. This program is layed out in such a way that anyone can do it. It is simple, yet challenging to the musculature.

IMPORTANT INFORMATION: How much strength to apply when performing these isometric contractions?Start off easy, then build. Contract the muscles by pulling and pushing with light to medium tension for the desired effect. As you progress, you may start pulling and pushing slightly harder but please not too hard. **Stimulate the muscles, do not annihilate them!**

How Should You Read This book? I recommend reading this book in its entirety before starting the exercise routines. There are some key elements that could be detrimental to your practice and your connective tissues if not done correctly. For example, holding your breath while doing isometrics could make you pass out, by increasing your blood pressure. The Power Iso-Bow Isometric Method is about mastering your muscle strength through your contraction.

What is Isometrics? Isometrics are exercises where your joints do not move. Normally with isotonic exercises, you move your joints through a full or partial range of motion. Lets look at a regular curl for example.You start off with the arm extended, then you slowly pull your arm upwards, then reverse the action. With an isometric exercise, you stay in a fixed position.

Isotonics and Isometrics Increase Muscle Size: There are loads of Isometric books on the market with 7 second contractions using excessive force suggesting it equals size increases. That's a fallacy and one of the main reasons muscle increases are very slow or most times non-existent for the masses that try isometric exercises in that manner. Hundreds of my students and friends have tried my methods, and they all receive massive growth spurts all of a sudden. **How?** They were neglecting the density method completely at every set of their workouts.

So exactly how can you activate those muscle-building dormant fibers to grow with Isometrics? The Power Iso-Bow Isometric Method are based on endurance with a density approach for enhancing growth factors because combining the two elements of endurance and density increases muscle-growth and the fat-burning process. This is caused by performing Isometric Power-Pulses, which extend the set you are focusing on. Stimulating both aspects of the endurance-oriented-2A fibers at each workout.

11/DEVELOP POWERFUL MUSCLES NOW

I've experienced fantastic gains in density and increased leaness, so have many of my trainees with my density specific methods. Extending time under load while combining strength and density within the workout is the best way of increasing muscle, burning fat and enhancing a lean physique.

Power-Pulses increases blood blockage as well as burning body-fat at an alarming rate. It is an excellent muscle-enhancing and conditioning tool, and I have used it exclusively as a teen and in my 20s on every exercise. The main reasons the methods works is that it allows you to reach the growth threshold without overtaxing your nervous system. Plus, without super heavy isometric contractions that place excessive trauma on joints and connective tissues.

So The truth of the matter is the growth threshold. This is the point at which the level of fatigue within the muscle is high enough that a growth response is ramped. Every isometric phase is aimed to fatigue the target muscles you are working, which ignites and tire all the various endurance 2As to promote muscle growth and strength gains. Now, lets get down to work......

Chapter 1:

CHEST

CREATE A RIPPED CHEST

CREATE A RIPPED CHEST

01 CREATE A RIPPED CHEST

The chest muscles allow you to push or move the arm forward or across the body. These muscles are activated in any throwing or pushing motion. Aesthetically, building a powerful chest is a sign of power in men.

However, the chest muscles are not used daily, so most times they are under developed. So despite, the simplicity of how these muscles contract, they can be trained in a number of various angles of push and pull, each offer its own special muscle enhancing properties.

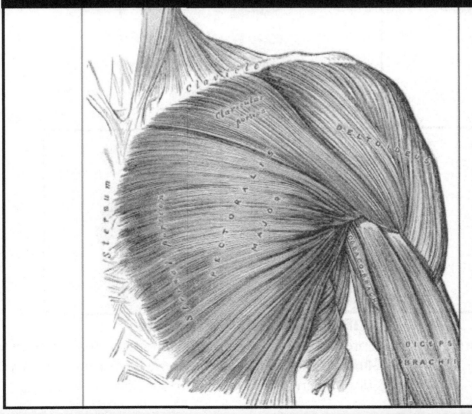

CHEST EXERCISES

01 CREATE A RIPPED CHEST

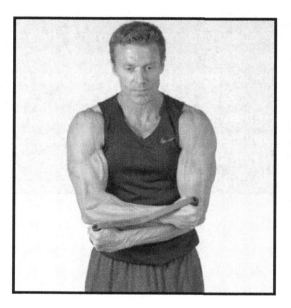

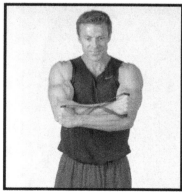
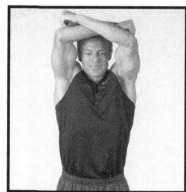

ISOMETRIC CHEST CONTRACTION

Cross arms as shown press the arms in opposite directions maintaining the tension. **(Isometric Contraction)** This exercise can be perform at various positions maintaining moderate tension.

Chapter 2:

SHOULDERS

DEVELOP RIPPED SHOULDERS

DEVELOP RIPPED SHOULDERS

02 DEVELOP RIPPED SHOULDERS

The shoulder muscles are divided into three heads and are quite unique and move the arm in all directions. The front muscle raise the arm forward, the side muscles made up of a number of muscle bundles, and raises the arm out to the sides. The rear or posterior muscle, is designed to pull the arm backwards. Forward raises is a peak contraction exercise. This exercise recruits the front and side heads of the shoulders that tie in well with stimulating the upper and mid-back muscles as well giving the entire girdle complete development.

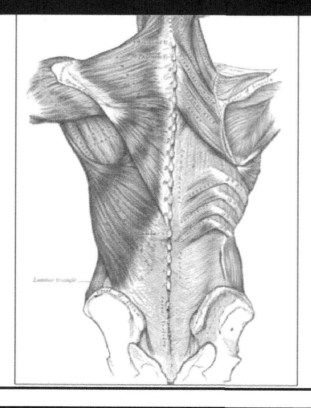

SHOULDER EXERCISES

02 DEVELOP RIPPED SHOULDERS

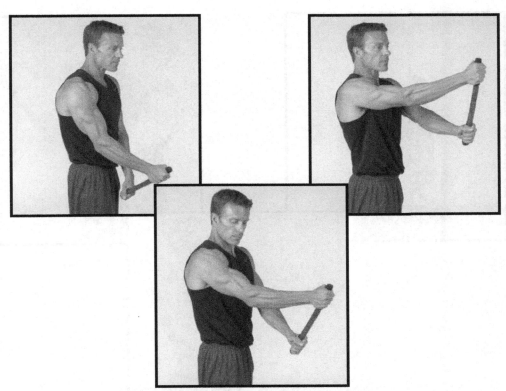

ISOMETRIC FORWARD CONTRACTION

Grasp the Iso-Bow in front of the body, as shown. We can do this movement at various angles for variety. Use moderate tension and keep breathing.
This works the front part of the shoulder muscles, along with the traps.

SHOULDER EXERCISES

02 DEVELOP RIPPED SHOULDERS

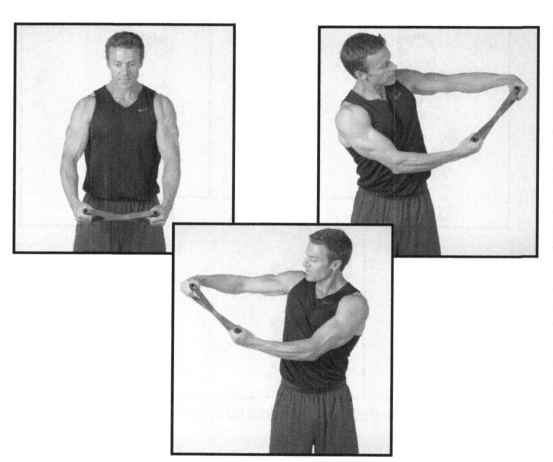

ISOMETRIC LATERAL RAISES

Hold the Iso-Bow at waist, keep your elbows slightly bent. We can do this movement at all three angles for variety. Use moderate tension and keep breathing.

SHOULDER EXERCISES

02 DEVELOP RIPPED SHOULDERS

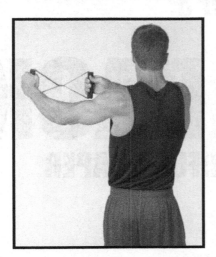 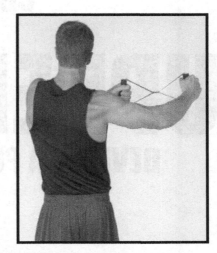

ACROSS THE BODY ISOMETRIC CONTRACTIONS

Place the Iso-Bow at chest height, keep your elbows slightly bent, pull Isometrically with the right hand while resisting with the other arm. Pause and reverse arms in opposite angle of pull.

Chapter 3:

UPPER BACK
DEVELOP A POWERFUL V-TAPER

DEVELOP A POWERFUL V-TAPER

03 DEVELOP A POWERFUL V-TAPER

The entire back is made up of many muscles overlapping each other. However, most trainees find the back quite difficult to fully develop. The reason? As the saying goes out of sight, out of mind. We cannot directly see the back muscles, plus we cannot see it flex like we would see the biceps.

We make training the entire back musculature much easier making developing the back obviously simple once you know what you are doing, you can bring these muscles up to speed. We are looking at the large Latissimus that covers the majority of the back. The trapezius is broken up into two sections.

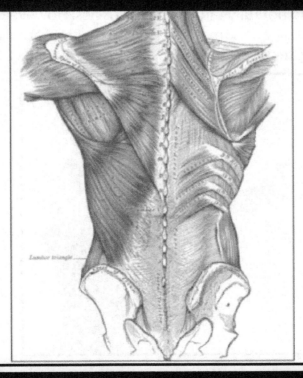

UPPER BACK EXERCISES

03 DEVELOP A POWERFUL V-TAPER

DO NOT NEGLECT THE MID AND LOWER TRAPS

The upper traps and mid-back muscles. Plus, we have the teres major, which is strongly stimulated with unilateral work, which makes isometrics the ideal movement. The infraspinatus muscle is like a half circle on each side of the upper back and is a very important rotator cuff muscle.

This muscle stabilizes the shoulder and prevents dislocations. Even though this muscle is at the back, most traditional exercises do not fully target these muscles. However, with our program there are Isometric exercises that target this area for full development.

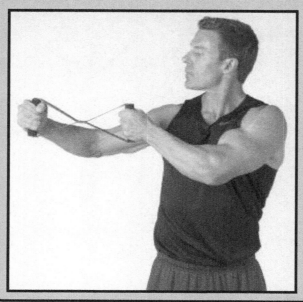

UPPER BACK EXERCISES

03 DEVELOP A POWERFUL V-TAPER

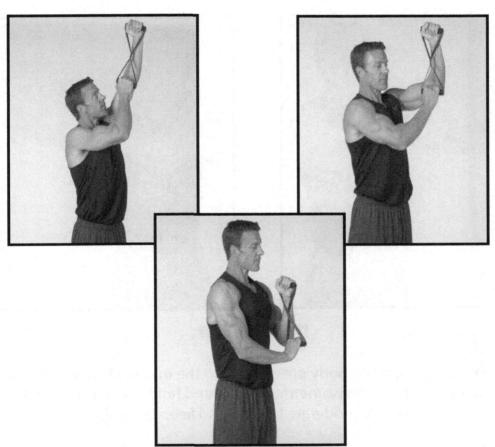

ISOMETRIC PULLDOWNS

Grasp the Iso-Bow as shown in the picture. This movement can be done at various angles for variety. Perform this action in an Isometric manner, use moderate tension and keep breathing

UPPER BACK EXERCISES

03 DEVELOP A POWERFUL V-TAPER

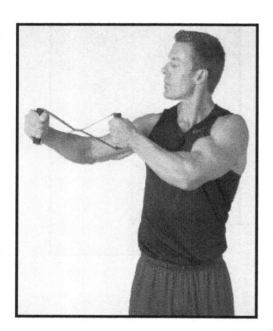 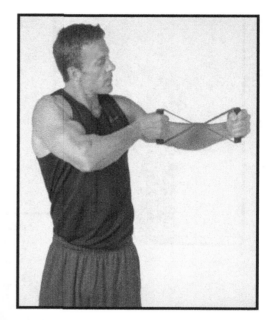

ISOMETRIC ROW

Bring your arm across the body pre-stretching the mid-back, grasp the Iso-Bow as shown. Pull in an Isometric manner and hold. Switch arms and continue. Use moderate tension and keep breathing

UPPER BACK EXERCISES

03 DEVELOP A POWERFUL V-TAPER

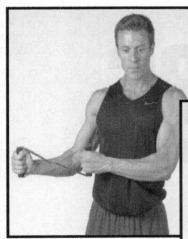
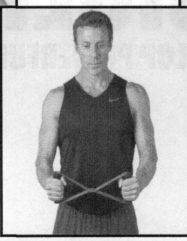
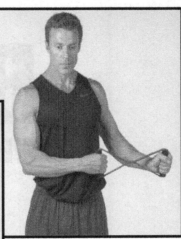

ADD POWER TO THE ROTATOR CUFF MUSCLES

Hold the Iso-Bow as shown. Pull with the left resisting isometrically with the right. This exercise can be done at various angles for variety. Use moderate tension and keep breathing

Chapter 4:

BICEPS

DEVELOP POWERFUL BICEPS

DEVELOP POWERFUL BICEPS

04 DEVELOP POWERFUL BICEPS

The biceps muscle has two heads. A short head, which is on the inside of the arm, and a long head, which is on the outside. This is the part that people see first. The main roll of the biceps is to flex the forearm by bringing the hand towards the shoulder. In order to build powerful complete biceps, you need to learn that the biceps do not work by itself.

The brachialis, which is under the bicep when developed, gives the bicep a larger and fuller appearance. Performing curls place undesirable tension on the tendon near the elbow. In other words, the biceps is placed in a very vulnerable position. Always start all bicep exercises with a slight bend at the start and finish. Always maintain tension on the biceps and not the joint.

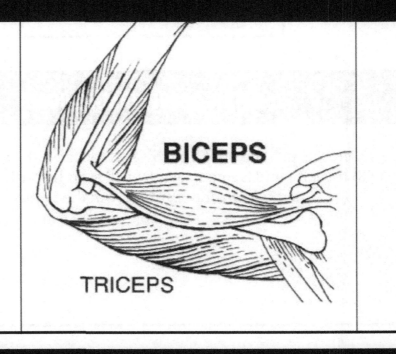

BICEP EXERCISES

04 DEVELOP POWERFUL BICEPS

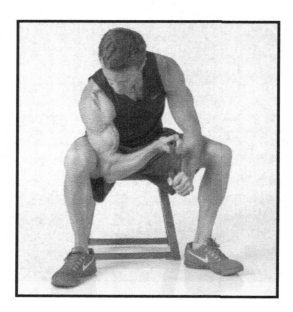

ISOMETRIC CONCENTRATION CURLS

As pictured, pull the right arm towards the face while resisting with the left hand Isometrically. Switch arms by pushing the left arm down and resisting with the right.

BICEP EXERCISES

04 DEVELOP POWERFUL BICEPS

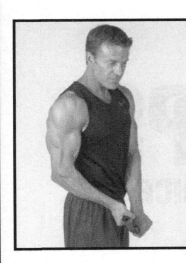 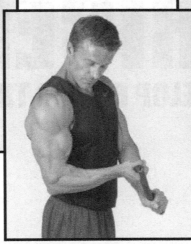 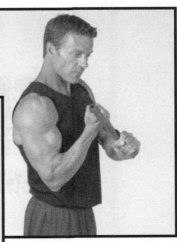

ISOMETRIC CURLS

Pull the right arm upward while resisting with the left hand Isometrically. Reverse arms and continue by pushing the left arm downwards, resisting with the right.

This movement can be done at various angles for variety. Use a moderate tension and keep breathing.

Chapter 5:

TRICEPS
DEVELOP RIPPED TRICEPS

DEVELOP RIPPED TRICEPS

05 DEVELOP RIPPED TRICEPS

DEVELOP RIPPED TRICEPS

The triceps has three heads: The lateral head, middle head and the long head. The role of the triceps is to straighten the arm. The triceps work in opposition to the biceps and brachialis muscles. The triceps has three heads this makes it much larger in mass than the biceps and the brachialis.

Unfortunately, most pay attention to the biceps, leaving the triceps underdeveloped. The lateral head, which is on the outside is what people see first. The triceps are easy to develop and we have made it easy for the trainee to achieve this.

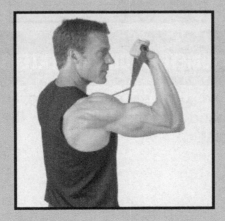

TRICEP EXERCISES

05 DEVELOP RIPPED TRICEPS

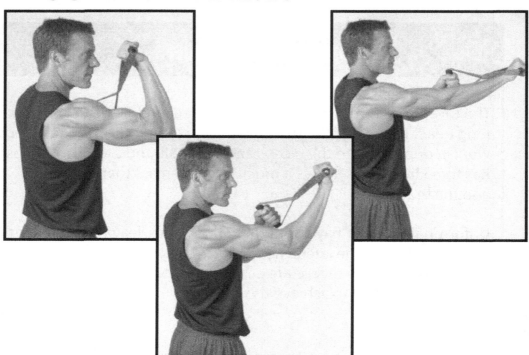

ISOMETRIC FORWARD EXTENSIONS

As shown above, push the right arm forward while resisting with the left hand at desired time frame **ISOMETRICALLY switch arms and repeat.**

TRICEP EXERCISES

05 DEVELOP RIPPED TRICEPS

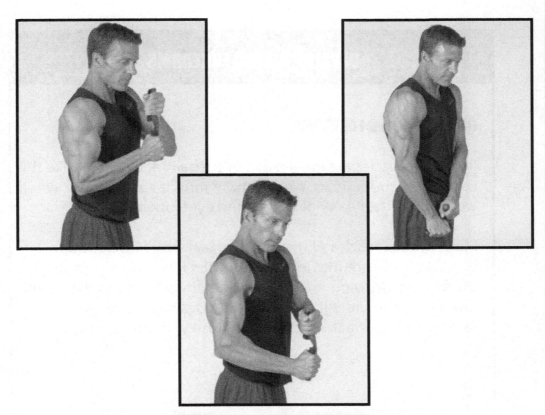

ISOMETRIC TRICEP PRESSDOWN

As pictured above, press the right hand downwards while resisting with the left arm. Change positions for variety. **RESIST ISOMETRICALLY**

DEVELOP RIPPED FOREARMS

06 DEVELOP RIPPED FOREARMS

DEVELOP RIPPED FOREARMS

DEVELOP RIPPED FOREARMS

Forearm muscles are involved in every daily activity, just like the calves and abdominals. We use these muscles all the time, when we drive, write, type, hold a bag and even open a door.

Many of the muscles of the forearm deal with Muscle-multi-use. When you are moving the elbow by lowering and raising the forearm. Moving the wrist up and down by, plus raising and lowering the hand. All Isometric exercises stress the forearms to contract which will increase your grip strength.

FOREARM EXERCISES

06 DEVELOP RIPPED FOREARMS

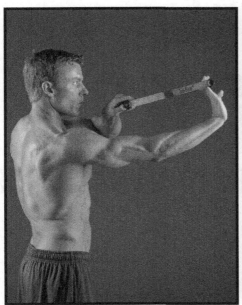
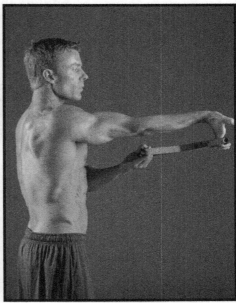

EXERCISE ONE   **EXERCISE TWO**

HAND/FOREARM EXERCISE

EXERCISE ONE: As pictured press the right hand forward. **RESIST ISOMETRICALLY and hold.**

EXERCISE TWO: Same as exercise one but, the hand is placed downwards.

Chapter 7:

THIGHS
DEVELOP POWERFUL TIRELESS THIGHS

DEVELOP POWERFUL TIRELESS THIGHS

07 DEVELOP POWERFUL TIRELESS THIGHS

DEVELOP POWERFUL TIRELESS THIGHS

The thigh muscles are basically made up of four main muscles: the vastus lateral muscle, this is located on the outside of the thighs. The vastus medial muscle, this is located on the inside of the thigh muscles towards the knee.

Better known as the tear drop because of its shape. The recus-femoris, which is located in the center of the muscles, and the vastus intermedius, this muscle is mostly covered by all the other muscles of the thighs. The Power Iso-Bow Isometric Method will develop tireless thighs with a power pack punch.

LEG EXERCISES

07 DEVELOP POWERFUL TIRELESS THIGHS

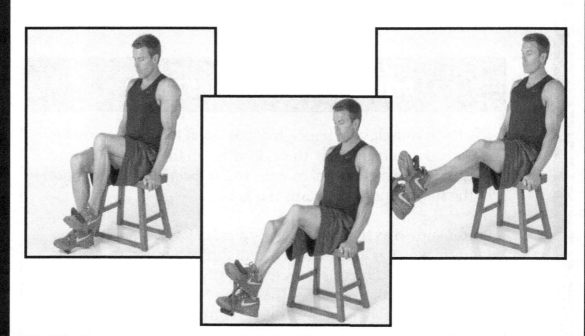

ISOMETRIC LEG EXTENSIONS

While seated on a chair, box or stool, place the legs as shown in the pictures. Maintain a Isometric static position for desired seconds, then switch legs. **RESIST ISOMETRICALLY**

LEG EXERCISES

07 DEVELOP POWERFUL TIRELESS THIGHS

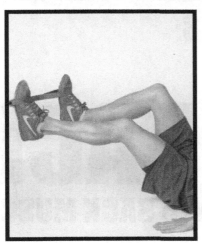 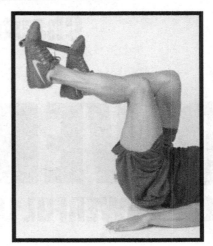

ISOMETRIC LEG PRESS

As shown, pull the right leg towards the chest, powerfully resisting with the left leg **Isometrically**. Switch legs and continue.

Chapter 8:

LOWER BACK
DEVELOP POWERFUL LOWER BACK MUSCLES

DEVELOP POWERFUL LOWER BACK MUSCLES

08 DEVELOP POWERFUL LOWER-BACK MUSCLES

POWERFUL LOWER BACK MUSCLES

Develop Powerful Lower back muscles

The lower back muscles support the lower part of the spine. When these muscles are well developed it builds a brace protecting the spine.

Apart from that the lower back muscles are responsible for bringing the body upright from a leaning forward position. Not only will the lower back be involved, but the glutes and hamstrings come into play.

LOWER BACK EXERCISES

08 DEVELOP POWERFUL LOWER BACK MUSCLES

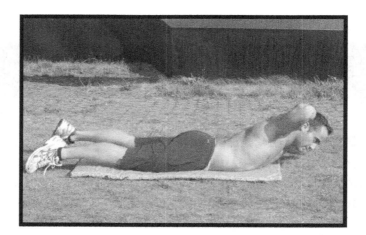

ISOMETRIC LOWER BACK EXTENSION

As shown above, lay flat on the floor and perform this movement by raising the upper body upwards and holding it Isometrically for the desired seconds.

Chapter 9:

CALVES
DEVELOP SHAPELY CALVES

DEVELOP SHAPELY CALVES

9 DEVELOP SHAPELY CALVES

DEVELOP SHAPELY CALVES

Develop shapely calves

The calves add a finished look to the lower leg with a diamond shape. This muscle has three heads (muscle parts) the soleus, this is under the large lateral head and gives the calves a fully developed look viewed from the side and back.

The lateral and medial heads are on the outside and in the middle of the muscle. The gastrocnemius make up the majority of the calf muscle. However, the longer the gastroc, the larger the potential for enhanced calf muscle development.

DEVELOP SHAPELY CALVES

9 DEVELOP SHAPELY CALVES

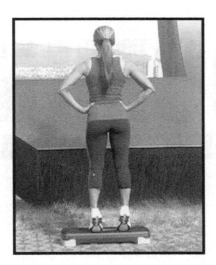

ISOMETRIC STANDING CALVE STANCE

Position yourself as shown but make sure the calves are contracted fully. Press straight up on the toes and hold the position Isometrically. This is a fantastic calve exercise.

Chapter 10:

ABDOMINALS
DEVELOP POWERFUL ABS

DEVELOP POWERFUL ABS

10 DEVELOP POWERFUL ABS

The abdominal muscles are very important and reveal that the trainee has a lean physique. Plus, the role of the abdominal muscles is to protect the spine. A lean chiseled set of abdominal muscles shows the opposite sex that the owner has a sign of virility.

Once these muscles are well developed this keeps the waist line and belly flat. There are various muscle structures that complete the overall look, the entire length of the abdominal wall, plus the internal and external obliques.

The lower sections of the abdominal muscles play the largest role in protecting the spine and storing belly fat. This is the easiest place for body-fat to accumulate. Which makes training with Isometric exercises ideal at stimulating those muscle fibers to the max.

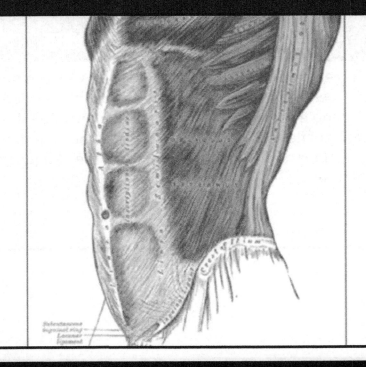

DEVELOP POWERFUL ABS

10 DEVELOP POWERFUL ABS

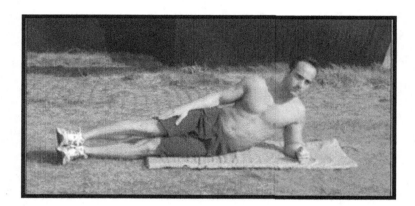

DEVELOP POWERFUL ABDOMINALS

As noted in the introduction the abdominal wall includes four muscles: Let's cover the entire length from the chest to pubis is called the rectus abdominis, people say abs for short. The abdominal wall should be worked in three angles of flexion. The lower sections of the abdominal muscles. The upper sections of the abdominal wall, and the obliques. Which are rotator muscles.

DEVELOP POWERFUL ABS

10 DEVELOP POWERFUL ABS

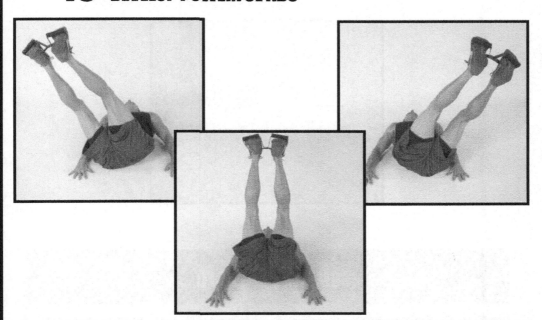

ISOMETRIC SIDE TO SIDE LATERAL RAISES

Normally people say I want to get rid of my love handles. This Isometric abdominal exercise really isolates the entire ab dominal way as well as the oblique muscles.

These muscles support the spine by making the abdominal wall more rigid. Start off as shown, spread the Iso-Bow apart maintaining Isometric tension. Try the movement at various angles as shown.

DEVELOP POWERFUL ABS

10 DEVELOP POWERFUL ABS

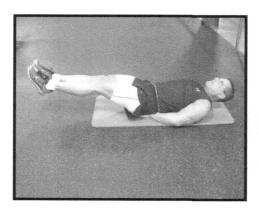

ISOMETRIC LEG HOLD

As shown above, place your hands under your butt and hold the position Isometrically for the desired seconds. This exercise stimulates the entire abdominal wall.

DEVELOP POWERFUL ABS

10 DEVELOP POWERFUL ABS

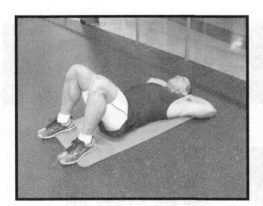 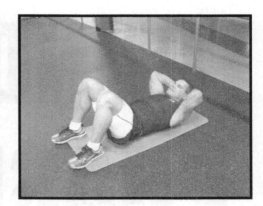

ISOMETRIC ABDOMINAL CRUNCHES

Lay on your back. Place the hands at your ear, tilt your head back, focus on the ceiling and go into the upward position as shown. **HOLD ISOMETRICALLY AND DO NOT PULL ON THE HEAD.**

Chapter 11:

FOUNDATION PHASE ONE

PERFORM EACH EXERCISE FOR 20 SECONDS, 3 SETS EACH BEFORE MOVING ONTO THE NEXT EXERCISE. REST 5 SECONDS BETWEEN SETS
ALL PHASES ARE TO BE PERFORMED FOR 2 WEEKS DO NOT SKIP PHASES

PHASE ONE

11 FOUNDATION

MONDAY, WEDNESDAY, FRIDAY

Perform 3 sets of 20 seconds each exercise. Perform each exercise using 50% of force. Rest 5 seconds between sets.

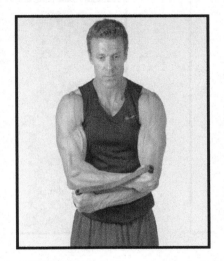

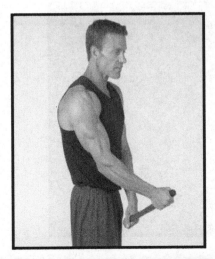
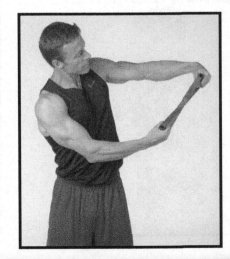

PHASE ONE

11 FOUNDATION

MONDAY, WEDNESDAY, FRIDAY
Routine continued.........

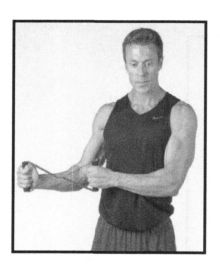

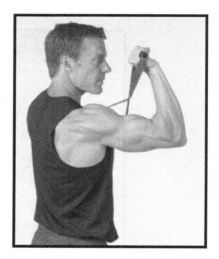

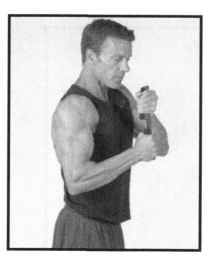

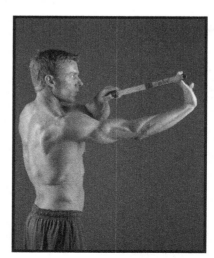

PHASE ONE

11 PHASE ONE

MONDAY, WEDNESDAY, FRIDAY
Routine continued...........

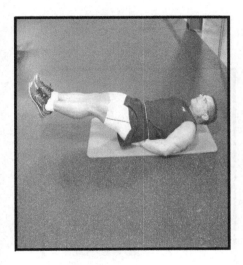 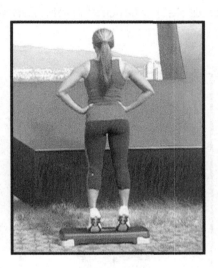

PHASE ONE MON, WED, FRI

PHASE ONE

11 PHASE ONE

TUESDAY, THURSDAY, SATURDAY

Perform 3 sets of 20 seconds each exercise. Perform each exercise using 50% of force. Rest 5 seconds between sets.

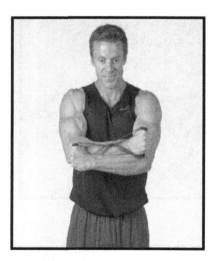
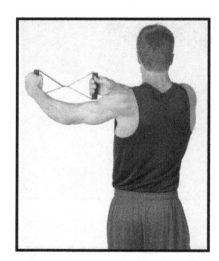
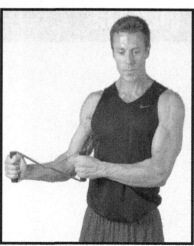
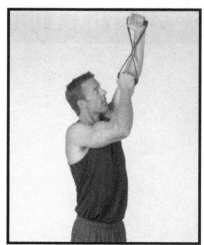

PHASE ONE

11 FOUNDATION

TUESDAY, THURSDAY, SATURDAY
Continued routine..........

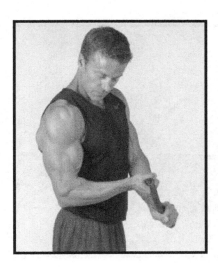
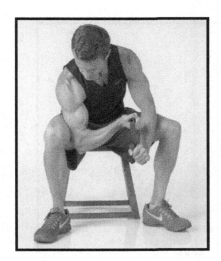

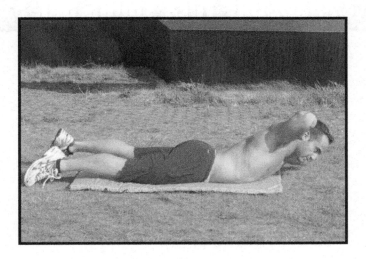

PHASE ONE

11 FOUNDATION

TUESDAY, THURSDAY, SATURDAY
Continued routine........

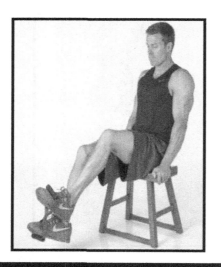 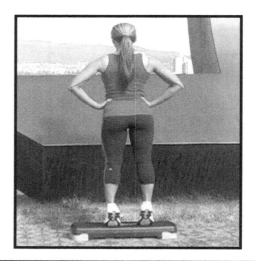

PHASE ONE TUES, THURS, SAT.

PHASE TWO

11 FOUNDATION X2

MONDAY, WEDNESDAY, FRIDAY

Perform 3 sets, 10 seconds before moving to the next exercise. Perform each exercise using 50% of force. Rest 5 seconds between sets.

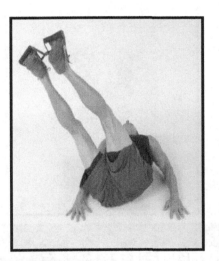
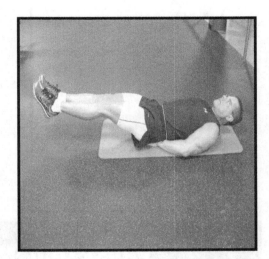

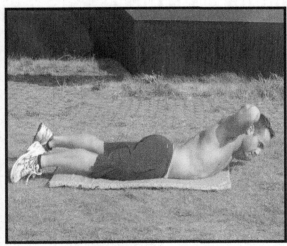
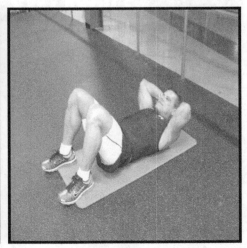

PHASE TWO

11 FOUNDATION X2

MONDAY, WEDNESDAY, FRIDAY
ROUTINE CONTINUED........

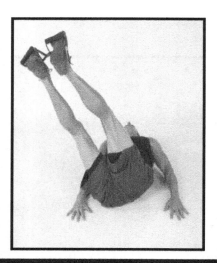
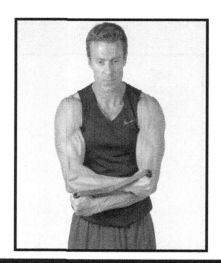

PHASE TWO   MON, WED, FRI.

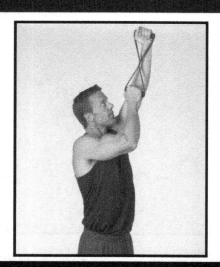
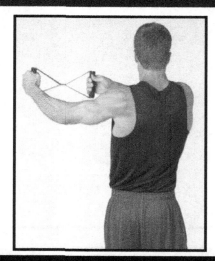

PHASE TWO

11 FOUNDATION X2

TUESDAY, THURSDAY, SATURDAY Perform 3 sets, 10 seconds each exercise before moving to the next exercise. Perform each exercise using 50% of force. Rest 5 seconds between sets.

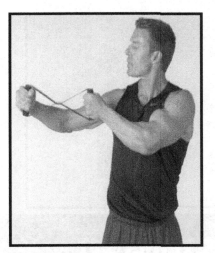

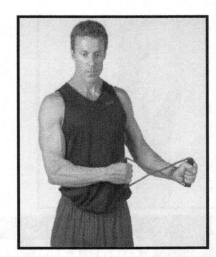

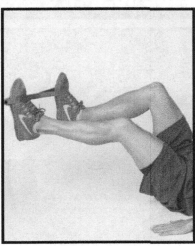

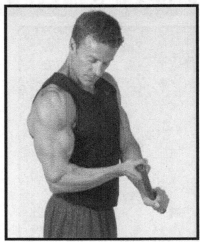

PHASE TWO

11 FOUNDATION X2

TUESDAY, THURSDAY, SATURDAY

ROUTINE CONTINUED..........

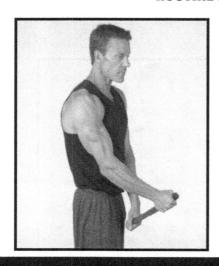 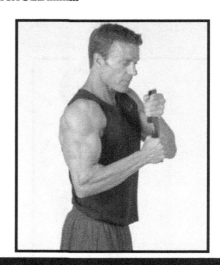

PHASE TWO   TUES, THURS, SAT.

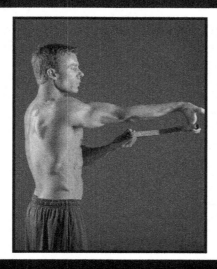 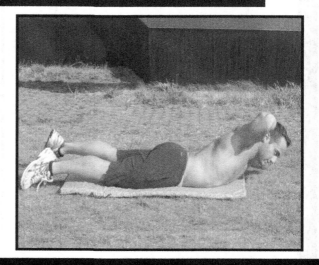

Chapter 12:

PHASE THREE

MUSCLE PUMP X3

ISOMETRIC LOAD TIME CHANGES WITHIN THE WEEK.
PERFORM PROGRAM 3 WEEKS

PHASE THREE

12 MUSCLE-PUMP X3

HOW TO PERFORM THIS ROUTINE:

Perform 2 sets, 40 seconds each exercise before moving to the next exercise. Perform each exercise using 50% of force. Rest 5 seconds between sets.

DAY ONE

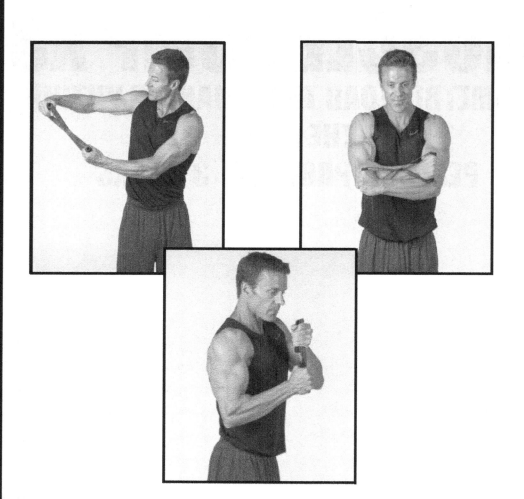

PHASE THREE

12 MUSCLE-PUMP X3

HOW TO PERFORM THIS ROUTINE:

Perform 2 sets, 40 seconds each exercise before moving to the next exercise. Perform each exercise using 50% of force. Rest 5 seconds between sets.

DAY ONE continued..........

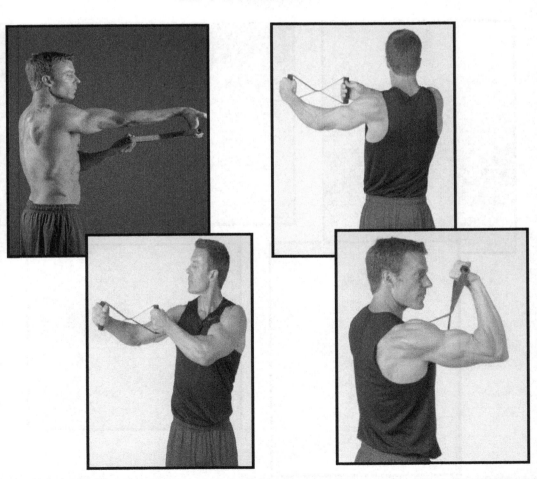

PHASE THREE

12 MUSCLE-PUMP X3

HOW TO PERFORM THIS ROUTINE:

Perform 2 sets, 40 seconds each exercise before moving to the next exercise. Perform each exercise using 50% of force. Rest 5 seconds between sets.

DAY TWO

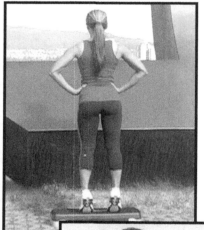

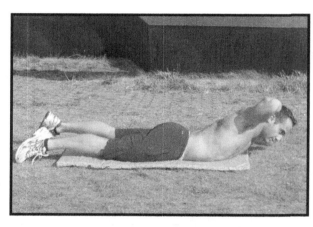

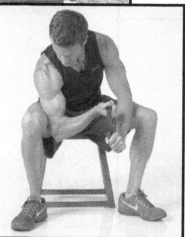

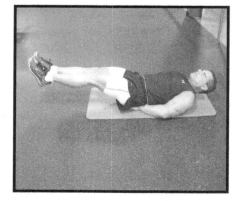

PHASE THREE

12 MUSCLE-PUMP X3

HOW TO PERFORM THIS ROUTINE:

Perform 2 sets, 40 seconds each exercise before moving to the next exercise.
Perform each exercise using 50% of force. Rest 5 seconds between sets.

DAY TWO continued..............

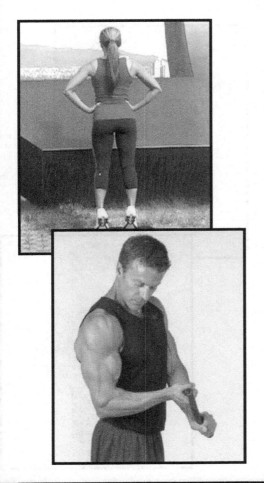

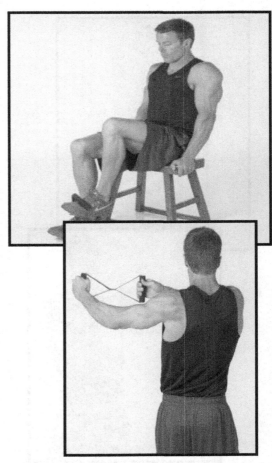

PHASE THREE

12 MUSCLE-PUMP X3

HOW TO PERFORM THIS ROUTINE:

Perform 4 sets, 15 seconds each exercise before moving to the next exercise. Perform each exercise using 50% of force. Rest 5 seconds between sets.

DAY THREE

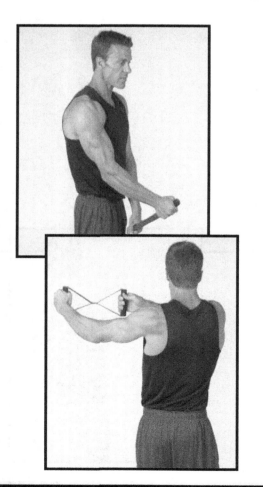

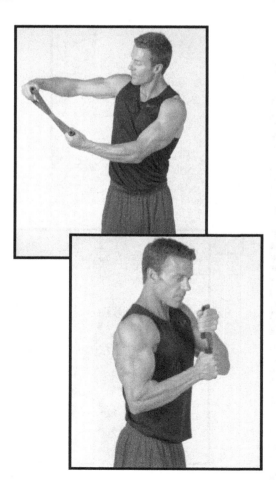

PHASE THREE

12 MUSCLE-PUMP X3

HOW TO PERFORM THIS ROUTINE:

Perform 4 sets, 15 seconds each exercise before moving to the next exercise. Perform each exercise using 50% of force. Rest 5 seconds between sets.

DAY THREE continued.......

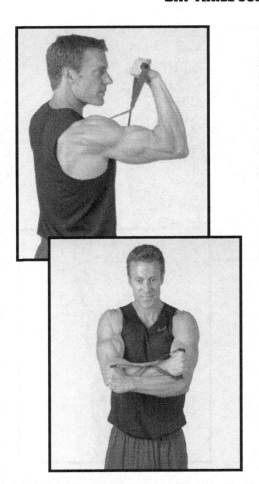

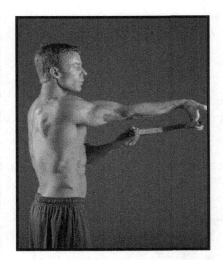

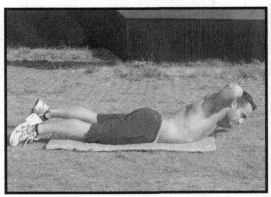

PHASE THREE

12 MUSCLE-PUMP X3

HOW TO PERFORM THIS ROUTINE:
Perform 4 sets, 15 seconds each exercise before moving to the next exercise. Perform each exercise using 50% of force. Rest 5 seconds between sets.

DAY THREE continued.......

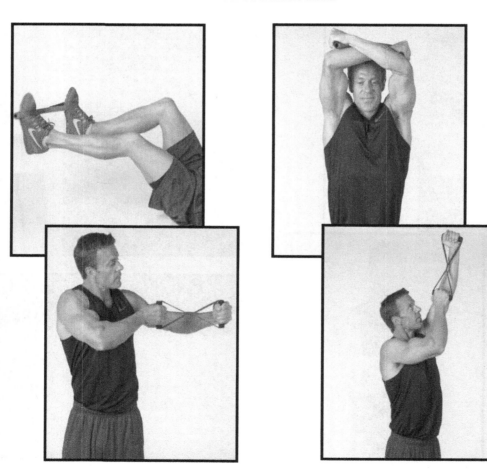

PHASE THREE

12 MUSCLE-PUMP X3

HOW TO PERFORM THIS ROUTINE:

Perform 3 sets, 50 seconds each exercise before moving to the next exercise. Perform each exercise using 50% of force. Rest 5 seconds between sets.

DAY FOUR

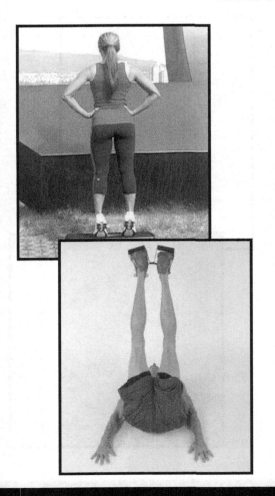

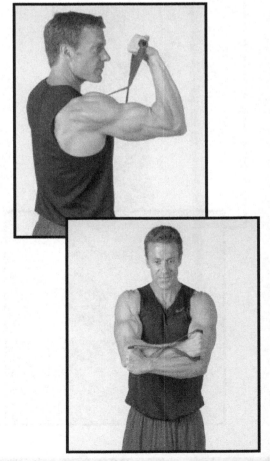

PHASE THREE

12 MUSCLE-PUMP X3

HOW TO PERFORM THIS ROUTINE:

Perform 3 sets, 50 seconds each exercise before moving to the next exercise. Perform each exercise using 50% of force. Rest 5 seconds between sets.

DAY FOUR continued......

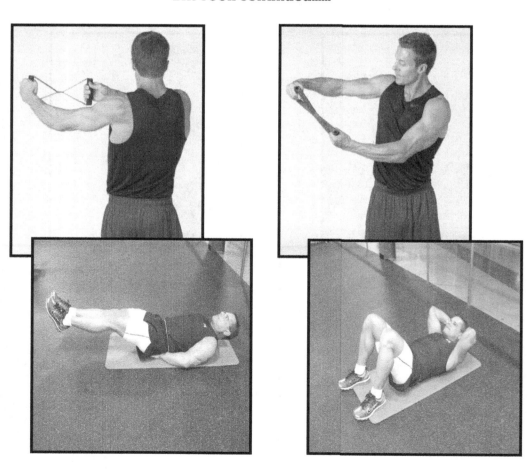

PHASE THREE

12 MUSCLE-PUMP X3

HOW TO PERFORM THIS ROUTINE:

Perform 3 sets, 30 seconds each exercise before moving to the next exercise. Perform each exercise using 50% of force. Rest 5 seconds between sets.

DAY FIVE

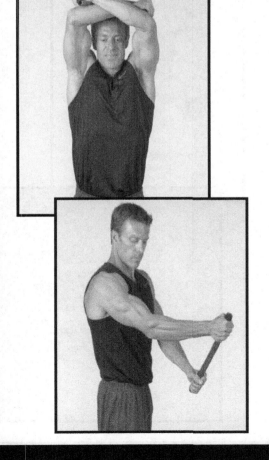

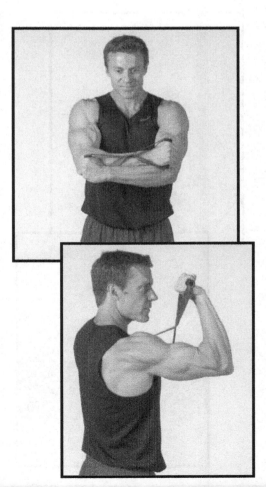

PHASE THREE

12 MUSCLE-PUMP X3

HOW TO PERFORM THIS ROUTINE:

Perform 3 sets, 30 seconds each exercise before moving to the next exercise. Perform each exercise using 50% of force. Rest 5 seconds between sets.

DAY FIVE continued.....

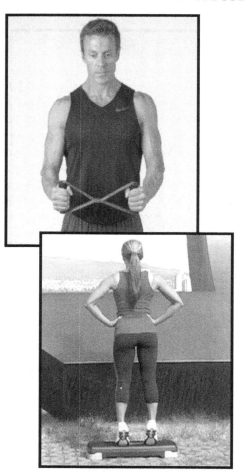

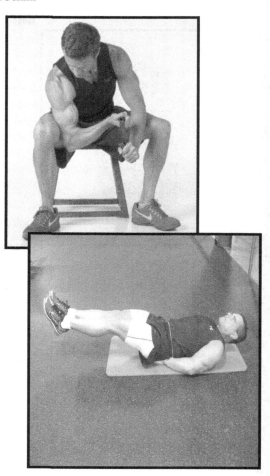

Chapter 13:

THE POWER X 20 MUSCLE-PULSE METHOD PHASE ONE

THE POWER X20 POWER-PULSE METHOD

13 THE POWER-PULSE METHOD

HOW TO PERFORM THIS ROUTINE:
PHASE ONE

Perform 20 one second Isometric pulses in reps style, followed by a 20 second Isometric contraction. Two sets per exercise. **CONTRACT ISOMETRICALLY FOR ONE SECOND, RELEASE AND CONTRACT AGAIN FOR DESIRED ISOMETRIC REPS**

DAY ONE

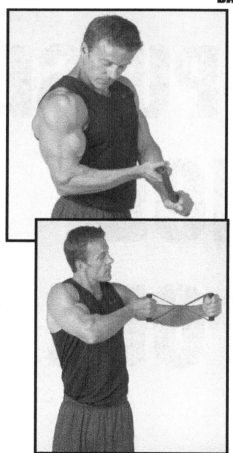
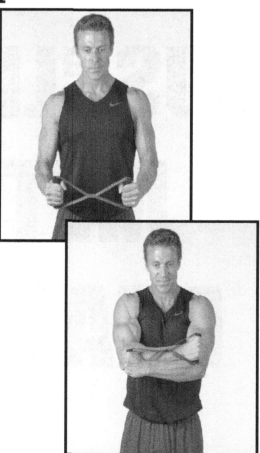

THE POWER X20 POWER-PULSE METHOD

13 THE POWER-PULSE METHOD

HOW TO PERFORM THIS ROUTINE:
PHASE ONE

Perform 20 one second Isometric pulses in reps style, followed by a 20 second Isometric contraction. Two sets per exercise. **CONTRACT ISOMETRICALLY FOR ONE SECOND, RELEASE AND CONTRACT AGAIN FOR DESIRED ISOMETRIC REPS**

DAY ONE continued............

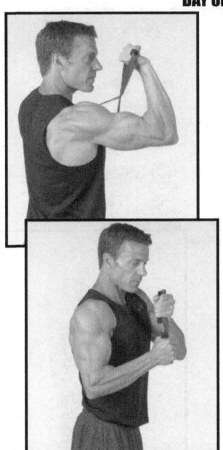

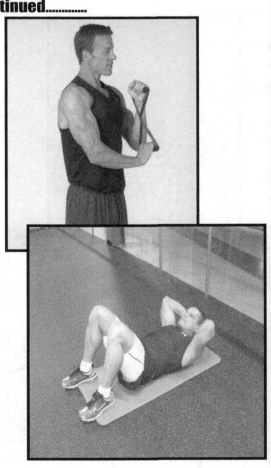

THE POWER X20 POWER-PULSE METHOD

13 THE POWER PULSE METHOD

HOW TO PERFORM THIS ROUTINE:
PHASE ONE

Perform 20 one second Isometric pulses in reps style, followed by a 20 second Isometric contraction. Two sets per exercise. **CONTRACT ISOMETRICALLY FOR ONE SECOND, RELEASE AND CONTRACT AGAIN FOR DESIRED ISOMETRIC REPS**

DAY TWO

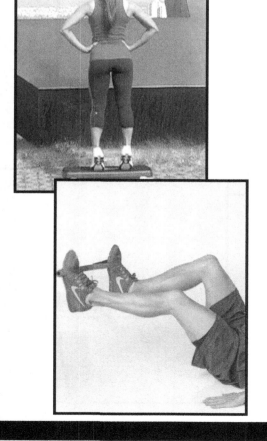
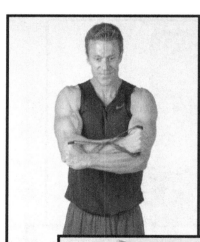
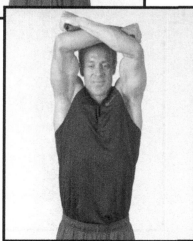

THE POWER X20 POWER-PULSE METHOD

13 THE POWER X20 POWER-PULSE METHOD

HOW TO PERFORM THIS ROUTINE:
PHASE ONE

Perform 20 one second Isometric pulses in reps style, followed by a 20 second Isometric contraction. Two sets per exercise. **CONTRACT ISOMETRICALLY FOR ONE SECOND, RELEASE AND CONTRACT AGAIN FOR DESIRED ISOMETRIC REPS**

DAY TWO continued.......

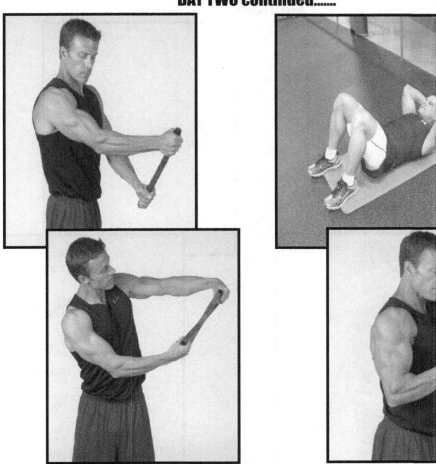

THE POWER X20 POWER-PULSE METHOD

13 THE POWER X20 POWER-PULSE METHOD

HOW TO PERFORM THIS ROUTINE:
PHASE ONE

Perform 20 one second Isometric pulses in reps style, followed by a 20 second Isometric contraction. Two sets per exercise. **CONTRACT ISOMETRICALLY FOR ONE SECOND, RELEASE AND CONTRACT AGAIN FOR DESIRED ISOMETRIC REPS**

DAY THREE

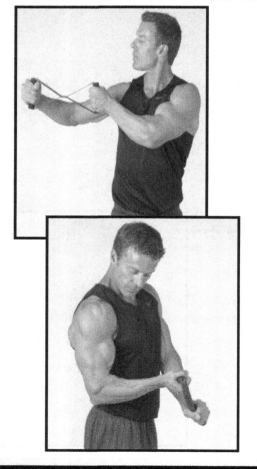

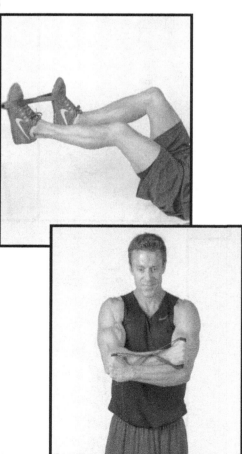

THE POWER X20 POWER-PULSE METHOD

13 THE POWER X20 POWER-PULSE

HOW TO PERFORM THIS ROUTINE:
PHASE ONE

Perform 20 one second Isometric pulses in reps style, followed by a 20 second Isometric contraction. Two sets per exercise. **CONTRACT ISOMETRICALLY FOR ONE SECOND, RELEASE AND CONTRACT AGAIN FOR DESIRED ISOMETRIC REPS**

DAY THREE continued..........

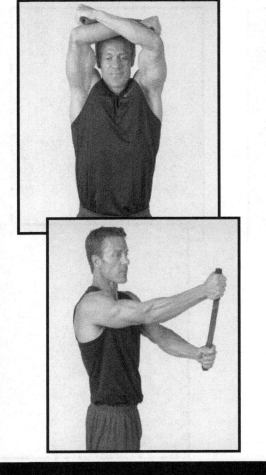

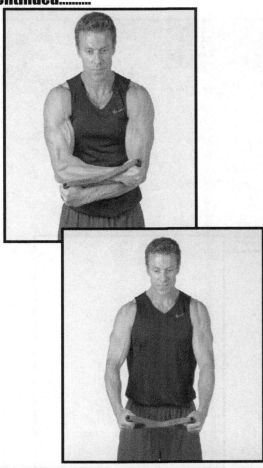

THE POWER X20 POWER-PULSE METHOD

13 THE POWER X20 POWER-PULSE

HOW TO PERFORM THIS ROUTINE:
PHASE ONE

Perform 20 one second Isometric pulses in reps style, followed by a 20 second Isometric contraction. Two sets per exercise. **CONTRACT ISOMETRICALLY FOR ONE SECOND, RELEASE AND CONTRACT AGAIN FOR DESIRED ISOMETRIC REPS**

DAY FOUR

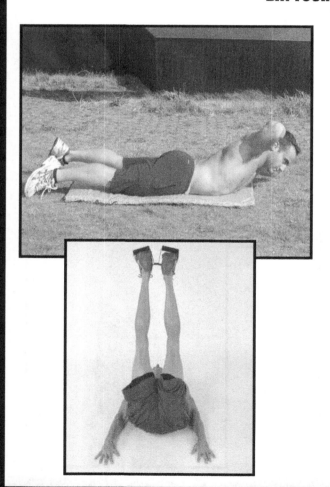

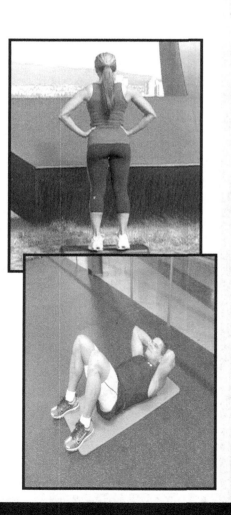

THE POWER X20 POWER-PULSE METHOD

13 THE POWER X20 POWER-PULSE METHOD

HOW TO PERFORM THIS ROUTINE:
PHASE ONE

Perform 20 one second Isometric pulses in reps style, followed by a 20 second Isometric contraction. Two sets per exercise. **CONTRACT ISOMETRICALLY FOR ONE SECOND, RELEASE AND CONTRACT AGAIN FOR DESIRED ISOMETRIC REPS**

DAY FIVE

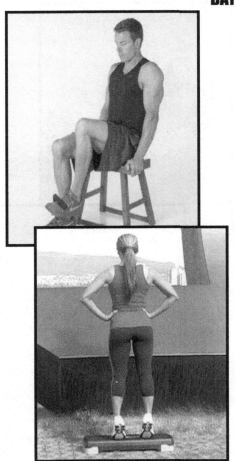

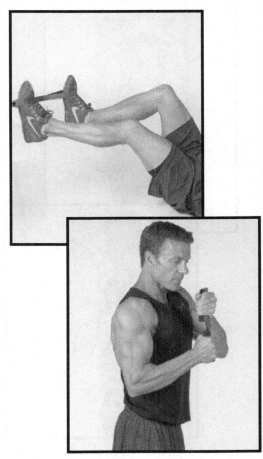

THE POWER X20 POWER-PULSE METHOD

13 THE POWER X20 POWER-PULSE METHOD

HOW TO PERFORM THIS ROUTINE:
PHASE ONE

Perform 20 one second Isometric pulses in reps style, followed by a 20 second Isometric contraction. Two sets per exercise. **CONTRACT ISOMETRICALLY FOR ONE SECOND, RELEASE AND CONTRACT AGAIN FOR DESIRED ISOMETRIC REPS**

DAY FIVE continued.............

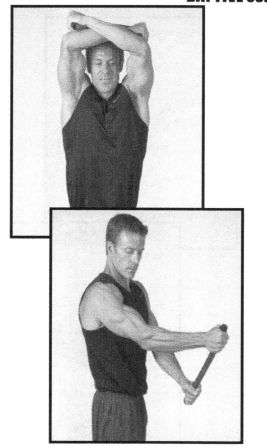

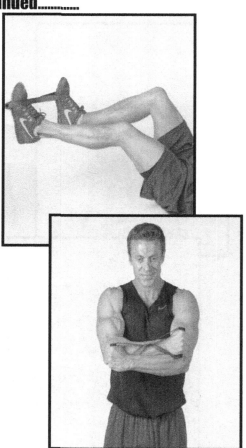

Chapter 13:

THE POWER X10 POWER-PULSE METHOD PHASE TWO

THE POWER X10 POWER-PULSE METHOD

13 THE POWER X10 POWER-PULSE METHOD

HOW TO PERFORM THIS ROUTINE:
PHASE TWO

Perform 10 one second Isometric pulses in reps style, followed by a 10 second Isometric contraction. Three sets per exercise. **CONTRACT ISOMETRICALLY FOR ONE SECOND, RELEASE AND CONTRACT AGAIN FOR DESIRED ISOMETRIC REPS**

DAY ONE

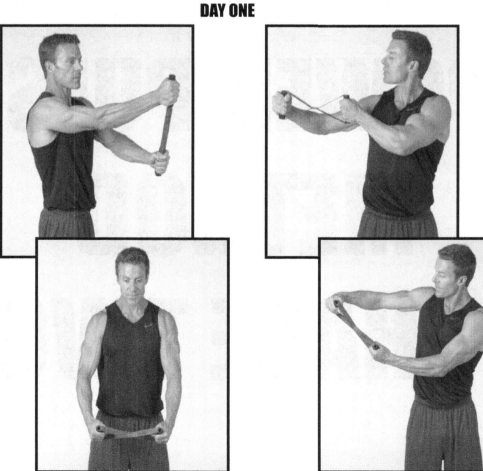

THE POWER X10 POWER-PULSE METHOD

13 THE POWER X10 POWER-PULSE METHOD

HOW TO PERFORM THIS ROUTINE:
PHASE TWO

Perform 10 one second Isometric pulses in reps style, followed by a 10 second Isometric contraction. Three sets per exercise. **CONTRACT ISOMETRICALLY FOR ONE SECOND, RELEASE AND CONTRACT AGAIN FOR DESIRED ISOMETRIC REPS**

DAY ONE continued..........

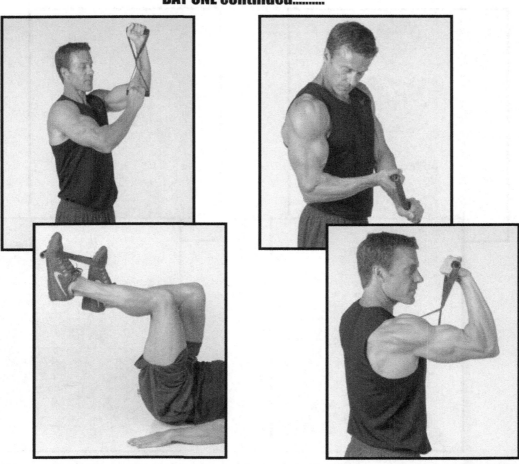

THE POWER X10 POWER-PULSE METHOD

13 THE POWER X10 POWER-PULSE METHOD

HOW TO PERFORM THIS ROUTINE:
PHASE TWO

Perform 10 one second Isometric pulses in reps style, followed by a 10 second Isometric contraction. Three sets per exercise. **CONTRACT ISOMETRICALLY FOR ONE SECOND, RELEASE AND CONTRACT AGAIN FOR DESIRED ISOMETRIC REPS**

DAY TWO

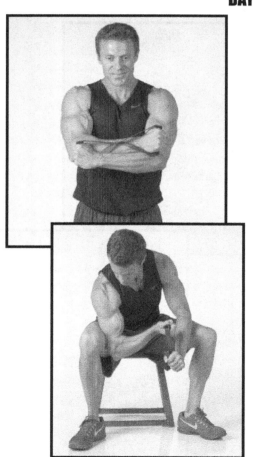

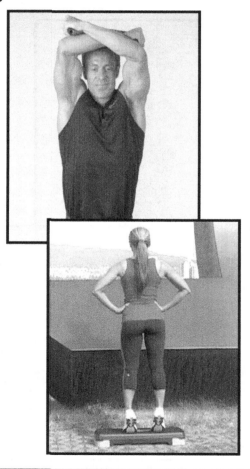

THE POWER X10 POWER-PULSE METHOD

13 THE POWER X10 POWER-PULSE METHOD

HOW TO PERFORM THIS ROUTINE:
PHASE TWO

Perform 10 one second Isometric pulses in reps style, followed by a 10 second Isometric contraction. Three sets per exercise. **CONTRACT ISOMETRICALLY FOR ONE SECOND, RELEASE AND CONTRACT AGAIN FOR DESIRED ISOMETRIC REPS**

DAY TWO continued........

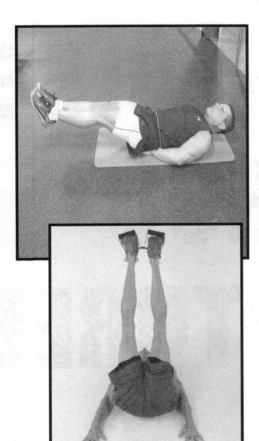
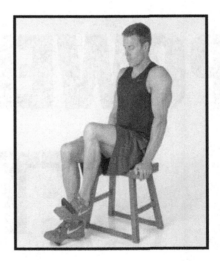
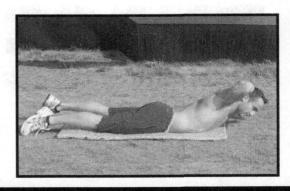

Chapter 13:

THE POWER X7 POWER-PULSE METHOD PHASE THREE

THE POWER X7 POWER-PULSE METHOD

13 THE POWER X7 POWER-PULSE METHOD

HOW TO PERFORM THIS ROUTINE:
PHASE THREE

Perform a 20 second isometric followed by 7 pulsing reps —each contraction lasting 2 seconds each. Alternate day one and day two for 6 days per week. Three sets each exercise, rest between 5 seconds.

DAY ONE

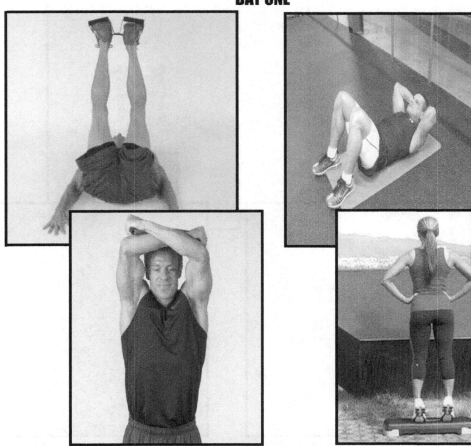

THE POWER X7 POWER-PULSE METHOD

13 THE POWER X7 POWER-PULSE METHOD

HOW TO PERFORM THIS ROUTINE:
PHASE THREE

Perform a 20 second isometric followed by 7 pulsing reps —each contraction lasting 2 seconds each. Alternate day one and day two for 6 days per week. Three sets each exercise, rest between 5 seconds.

DAY ONE continued............

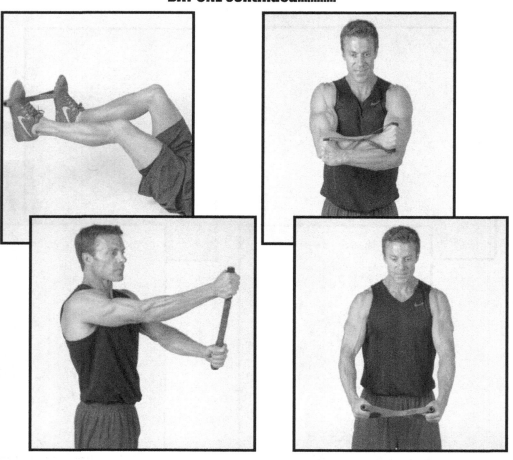

THE POWER X7 POWER-PULSE METHOD

13 THE POWER X7 POWER-PULSE METHOD

HOW TO PERFORM THIS ROUTINE:
PHASE THREE

Perform a 20 second isometric followed by 7 pulsing reps —each contraction lasting 2 seconds each. Alternate day one and day two for 6 days per week. Three sets each exercise, rest between 5 seconds.

DAY TWO

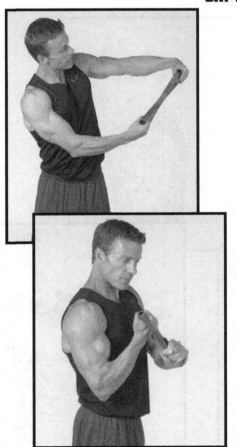

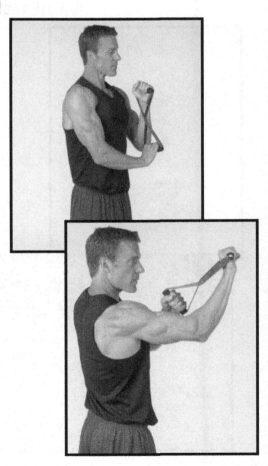

THE POWER X7 POWER-PULSE METHOD

13 THE POWER X7 POWER-PULSE METHOD

HOW TO PERFORM THIS ROUTINE:
PHASE THREE

Perform a 20 second isometric followed by 7 pulsing reps —each contraction lasting 2 seconds each. Alternate day one and day two for 6 days per week. Three sets each exercise, rest between 5 seconds.

DAY TWO continued...........

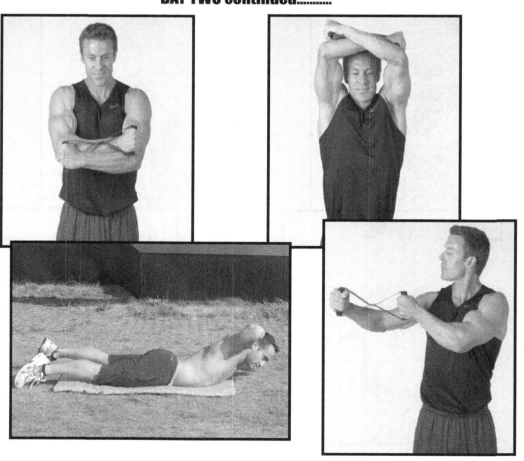

We are looking forward to hearing from you on your progress. Please drop us an email skippymarl@icloud. com

Made in the USA
Middletown, DE
21 August 2022

71902129R00057